DISMANTLING
Anxiety

DISMANTLING Anxiety

GAIL BENNETT FRY

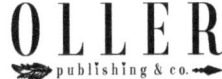

Duped: Dismantling Anxiety
Copyright © 2023 by Gail Bennett Fry
Cover and Layout Design by Cheryl Chaney

All rights reserved. No part of this book may be reproduced or transmitted in any form or by any means without written permission from the author.

God has brought us together.
You, me. For such a time as this...

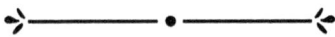

Please note: There has been no editing by the publisher in the content of this book, solely at the author's request. Gail wanted her words to appear exactly as she wrote them. From her heart to her hand to her tablet, complete with any and all imperfections.

I remember that day….sitting in the doctor's office. Just an ordinary checkup. Nothing unusual. Nothing suspect. I checked myself in at the front reception desk and headed for the waiting room. What a clever name: **Waiting Room**. Certainly lives up to its title because you go there to wait and wait and wait!! Now this was just before smartphones had been permanently affixed to the palm of our hand, to either entertain, inform, or distract us, whatever the case may be. Either way, you always have something to keep you busy and not think about how long you have been sitting there. SO, after I had flipped through every magazine in the room and being quite sure that neither Fishing or Popular Mechanics was something I would ever choose to pursue, I happened to spot a nearby table with some loose fliers on it. "Let's go take a look" I thought to myself. "What does this say? Something about Anxiety and if left untreated can lead to Chronic Anxiety.

Hmm…." I began to read all of the negative things anxiety can do to your body, immune system and pretty much everything else that is important to you in your life. Then it starts listing all the ways to keep anxiety at bay and one of them is keeping stress out of your life. **"Yeah!! That's easy!!"** I say to myself very sarcastically. "Who wrote this article anyway?!" Thankfully I hear my name being called and **eagerly** return the flier to its original spot all the while thinking how lucky that I had dodged **that** bullet and none of that information pertained to me…..

Okay, I want to hit the Pause button for a minute. Please stay with me. I promise I am not going off the grid. I will give you clarity in just a minute.

Who knows what a termite is? For those of you who don't, let me quickly give you a definition. A termite is a very small insect with a ravenous, insatiable appetite for wood. They are found on every continent except Antarctica. They travel in huge colonies and are devastatingly destructive to homes. They can literally eat away the foundation and interior framing of a home or building causing it to collapse. You know what their biggest advantage is? They go **undetected.** They are usually never seen until the destruction has been completed. All you have left is pulverized pulp.

Okay, let's push the Play button again and proceed. I'll tie all this information together and give you the clarity I promised. The reason I wanted you to know about termites is because Anxiety and termites have a lot in common. Anxiety also goes undetected and does just what the termite does. It hollows a person out and leaves a vicious venom behind, **FEAR**, to fill the void it has created. It, too, has an insatiable appetite. Anxiety termites are sneaky dangerous. I am living proof of this. Remember that flier I told you about earlier in my doctor's office? Well, Anxiety termites were working on me at that very moment and had been for a good part of my life. I had not detected them until a few months later when **MY** house collapsed and I almost reached the point of no return. I was riddled with Anxiety termites. I was forced to rebuild. And I learned that you cannot rebuild with the damaged, termite ridden wood. You have to introduce new, healthy wood. I am here to tell you how to build back. To give you tools. You will need them desperately to build back correctly and safeguard your house for the future.

It's often a mystery as to what, when, how and why anxiety starts to inhabit an individual. Anxiety is non-discriminatory. It attacks people of all age, gender, race, intelligence, health, wealth and economic situations. I could recite hundreds of very valid reasons as the cause of anxiety but I can assure you this; there is only one way out. You **have** to go back to where it all began….in your mind.

Please. Come sit with me for a while.

Gail

"**S**o... I see you're looking for a magic wand", said the pretty, fiftyish blonde therapist sitting directly across from me. "**What?!!** What did she just say?!! You have got to be kidding me!! Well, this is just great! I get a Whack-O right out of the gate! Just my luck. Here I am, a grown woman and this girl is talking about fairy tales, which by the way, my life has been anything **BUT** for a good long while. "You're the doctor, **FIX ME!!!**" I say to myself. Just moments earlier I had poured out my heart and emptied my head, or what I had left, to this woman, who I very affectionately **NOW**, call Jan. I was in trouble, and I knew it. So did everybody else. Months earlier I had developed a serious health issue which sent me down a rabbit hole. **DAMN**. Not again. I was familiar with rabbit holes. I had fallen in one in 1991 when I lost my beautiful 15 year old daughter, Jamie, in an automobile accident. But this one was different. This one would have sent Bugs Bunny himself running to the medicine cabinet for anything he could lay his hands on. And this time he did....Grief is very different from Anxiety. Grief is full of despair, sadness, anger and hopelessness. Anxiety is **FEAR**. Plain and simple. Okay, I want to stop here for just a second and say something about the word you just heard me say a moment ago, damn. Yes, I saw you rolling your eyes, wondering how much profanity this girl was going to use. I can assure you, not much. But sometimes profanity is necessary. For me, the word damn is the expression of something very intense. I want you to **KNOW** that. **FEEL** that. There is a very famous chocolatier who labels his chocolate as Intense Dark Chocolate. Now stay with me for a minute. I have been involved in the homebuilding and interior design industry over the years and you quickly learn that the word "quaint" is code for old and the word "cozy" is code for small. So in Gail Fry's lexicon, the word "intense" is code for damn. So, what that chocolatier is really trying to tell you is "Damn, that's good chocolate!" I would even go as far as to say that I think damn should be considered an adjective! Wait for it… Wait for it…**BAM!!** "Did you just hear that loud thud?" That was every English teacher across America falling out of their chairs!! Seriously, words are very important and the basis or groundwork for our learning process.

And, man oh man, have I learned a lot over the past five years about a subject that I wished I had no knowledge of, Anxiety. **STILL** learning. Remember that magic wand my friend Jan talked about earlier? Well, I've been looking for it all this time and at this writing have yet to locate it. **BUT** in my search I have learned some very valuable knowledge that I think might help you. Please. Take my hand. I will hold on very tight and together you and I will make it through this. I promise.   Gail

"Why does my brain hate me?" I would ask that question week after week to Jan. The brain is absolutely fascinating and I am in complete and total **AWE** that God has entrusted me with this beautiful, powerful piece of machinery. Your brain is very much like a computer and **YOU** are the computer programmer. That's a lot of responsibility!! **NEWS FLASH**!! Bill Gates is not the first to build a computer, God is!! Whether you realize it or not, everything you experience with any of your senses--sight, sound, smell, taste and touch registers in that beautiful computer sitting on top of your shoulders and produces a thought or opinion which drives our actions. Memory is a key player in all of this too, but we'll talk about him later. Isn't it so cool when you are trying to think of something, a song or a person's name, and at that moment you can't recall it so you give up and go on to something else. Then later, when you have totally forgotten about it, the answer suddenly pops into your brain! So cool! Your brain never stopped searching for the answer to your question. It keeps searching all the files in your head until it locates it and delivers it right to you. Talk about an awesome search engine!! But, if not well taken care of, it too is vulnerable to bugs, viruses and ransom. The Bible warns us many, many times about guarding our minds.

For a very long time I mistakenly blamed my innocent brain for all of my troubles. It took me a long time to admit that it was not my brain that was the villain but it was the girl sitting at the keyboard to my brain that was confused. I had to fire her. But before her departure she had done **A LOT** of damage. I was a trainwreck. I was diagnosed with GAD, generalized anxiety disorder. And for those who know me well, are already aware of my battle with OCD, obsessive compulsive disorder. **HOLY NIGHTMARE BATMAN!!!** One more acronym and my head will explode!!

I am sitting here today having this conversation with you after many hours of hard work, tears, prayers and a **BIG** dose of reality. I credit Jan Kimball, my therapist, with literally saving my life. But I was a very good student and am still learning. The first step to getting better is admitting that something has to change and that is your view of things. Your perception. In the beginning of my therapy I was given a list of ten unhealthy thinking patterns that I probably was guilty of. Ya think?!! I fought it vehemently. Not me!! No way!! I look at these now and oh my gosh!!!! I practiced them all!! They were so ingrained in my thinking. They were habits. It's very hard work to change unhealthy habits but oh my gosh, so worth it!! Anxiety is like cancer. It grows silently within you until one day it surfaces its ugly head and you have to confront it. When it took the form of physical symptoms is when I finally took action. I could no longer function as a healthy, independent adult.

It doesn't matter how you got here, dear friend. We are in the same boat. You CAN get better. I'm living proof. The way I see it is you have two choices. (1) You can stop this conversation right now and totally disregard everything I want to share with you AND stay on the same road you are traveling or (2) You can turn the page. Hope to see you on the other side.

While you weren't looking, your unsupervised brain wandered out onto the street and hooked up with some pretty shady characters. They seemed innocent enough at the time. How were you to know? You began to learn what I call 'Trash Talk' from them. The medical community calls it cognitive distortions but I'm going to call it Trash Talk from here on out, because that's exactly what it is. Your brain starts having a steady diet of this kind of talk which translates into your way of thinking which translates into your behavior which more often than not turns into anxiety. It becomes a habit very quickly when this kind of thinking is the only thing on the menu. You have got to be honest with yourself and consider the possibility that maybe this has become your steady diet. It was okay for a while but now you have crashed. Some of you will never even consider talking with a therapist for a variety of reasons which I totally understand and respect. This is why I want to talk to you. Give you the valuable, life saving information given to me, in my own words. Show you that you are not the only one that feels the way you do. Give you a plan. Let's get started.

Admission

Admitting that you even **HAVE** anxiety is very difficult. It was for me. It was only until I started experiencing physical symptoms in my body that I started to believe that I was the victim of anxiety. I made one trip to the Emergency Room convinced I was having a heart attack. Nada. The fact that you and I are even having this conversation is **HUGE!!** Please don't discount the significance of this. You have to recognize who your enemy is. It is anxiety. It is **NOT** you, my friend. Very quietly, an uninvited intruder crept into your brain with stealth-like agility and unpacked his bags. He very methodically filled every nook and cranny of storage space he could find. *He went through your underwear drawer.* You never felt a thing. Until now. But good news, my friend! The enemy now has a face! His identity has been compromised! **NOW** we can learn to fight!

Consistency/Routine

Our brains like consistency. Ever hear of circadian rhythms? These are 24 hour cycles that are part of the body's internal clock. We've all heard of the sleep-wake cycle. This is a circadian rhythm. God is so cool. He created our brains to adapt and handle spontaneity and crisis but He wants us to feel safe. Safe is good for an anxious person and consistency, routine and structure is crucial to this. I know you've heard it a million times before, but going to bed and getting up at the same time every day is very good for your brain and well being. It craves it. Just like food, water and exercise is crucial for your body to operate optimally, sleep is **HUGE** for your brain! You truly do have an internal clock and it craves continuity to perform optimally. God is very consistent. Have you ever experienced a day without a night? Has the ocean ever had a high tide without a low tide? When you take in a breath, inhale, you automatically breathe out, exhale. Consistency may sound very mundane to some and some may think this practice would stifle or suppress their creativity but actually it's quite the opposite. When the brain is not being taxed with tasks undone or worry about uncertainty of things to come, it frees the brain to soar into realms of calm and creativity. Einstein wore the same type of clothing everyday. Consistency. Let it work for you.

Perseverance

"You are running a marathon, not a sprint." Jan said this to me over and over again. **NOT** what I wanted to hear!! Yuk!! Remember when we first started talking and I told you about my first visit to Jan? I wanted her to **FIX ME?!** I looked for that stupid magic wand for years. You so badly want to go back to your previous life. Life without experiencing the effects of anxiety. We live in such a microwave society. Everything comes quickly without much effort. But as we grow and mature, we learn that is not always the case. When you want to lose weight it takes time. You cannot merely think about losing weight, you have to put the effort, discipline and time that it takes to accomplish this goal. Same thing for building a house, letting your hair grow, planting a garden, learning a new language, etc. The key is to **NOT** get discouraged. From the very first meeting with Jan she had me bring a spiral notebook to every visit. And since I am the **ULTIMATE** rule follower, I did! I would write down everything I was experiencing and she would give me advice and sometimes homework. I **CHERISH** my notebook!! The first pages of my notebook my handwriting is huge, all over the page because my hand was so shaky back then. I would ask the same questions over and over. But as time went by my handwriting became smaller, more legible. More coherent. Step by step I was getting better. But it took a long time. I'm **STILL** working at it! Probably always will be, but **OH MY GOSH!!** I am so much better!! I am living again!! I have tools to help me! Please, put your running shoes on! You can do this! It is **SO** worth it! There will be days that you just have to stop and take a rest and that's **OKAY!!** It will not erase all the progress you've made. Don't let your enemy fool you into that frame of mind. Create your own mantra. You **WILL** reach your goal.

Be Kind to Yourself

This was **VERY** hard for me. "You are such a hard taskmaster!" Jan would say to me, right from the very beginning. What?!! What does that even mean?! I was the girl who didn't even need to have real enemies because I was my worst. True story. I took responsibility for **EVERYTHING!!!** I was a mean girl, but only to myself. I grew up being a people pleaser which everyone knows only works half the time!! When I would make a mistake I would loathe myself. Well, I am happy to tell you that I divorced that girl and my only regret is that I didn't do it a lot sooner!! Seriously, this is major stuff. I had to **PRACTICE** learning how to be nice to myself. I know it sounds crazy, but it's true. Some of you probably know exactly what I'm talking about. I was always the first to point out my flaws and weaknesses. I always wanted to make sure people knew that I knew about them. How sad. This is one of the many practices that helped create my anxiety. When you finally figure out that you are a valuable person worthy of love and respect from others **AND** yourself you will gain unbelievable confidence! Not cocky confidence that nobody likes, but empowering confidence. We'll talk more about this later but I want you to know that when you become able to recognize and defeat all of this Trash Talk you will experience confidence like you've never had before. **HELLO WORLD!!!**

Remember earlier when we talked about how your senses; sight, sound, smell, taste and touch register an immediate thought, opinion or memory in your brain? All within a nanosecond! Well, I believe the smartest guy in the room (brain) or at least the one who holds the most influence, is Memory. Your memory is the guy who is observing and recording everything your brain is experiencing. He writes down your opinion and reaction to what you are seeing, hearing, smelling, tasting and feeling whether it's good, bad or ugly, right or wrong, rational or irrational. This is all for future reference to be used for decision making in the future. Pretty cool, huh? Memory, I believe, is the most valuable gift God has given us. Don't you just love it when you see something or someone that triggers a beautiful memory? Or hear a song that takes you back to High School? Or smell the fragrance of your mom's cologne? Or taste the homemade chicken pot pie your grandma used to make? Or the touch of your first kiss? The beautiful gift of Memory is what enables me to spend wonderful time with my beautiful daughter since I am temporarily no longer able to, in the physical sense. I can walk through wonderful memories in my mind and see her beautiful smile, feel her hugs, hear her laughter. There are no words to describe how valuable these memories are to me. Thank you Lord Jesus for the gift of Memory. Wow. We rely on memory to help us make decisions everyday. It is a very valuable asset. It is this beautiful gift that saves time so we don't have to learn and relearn things over and over again. It makes information already learned readily available.

Memory is a Historian. It is the news reporter and news anchor. Everything needs to be recorded, right? For future reference, right? There's only one problem with this. We're Human and guess what? Sometimes humans don't always perceive things rationally. I want to give you an example. When I was about 6 years old I was attacked and bitten by a ferocious Red Chow dog. This happened at a friend's house who owned Chows. My father was also attacked while heroically trying to save me. Thank you Daddy. This event terrified me. Prior to this event I absolutely loved dogs, well puppies. Sadly, we lived on a very busy street and most of our dogs never made it to adulthood! But I never recall any fear of them. Well, after this event, guess who is terrified of dogs?!! You guessed it. Me. Now stay with me on this. I want to introduce you to a **new** little character in our brain. He is called the amygdala. This little guy's job is to come out with his hair on fire screaming, "Run! Run for your life! The sky is falling!!" when you experience a life threatening event or danger of some sort, real or imagined. You need to look up all the things your body and brain does to prepare itself for either a fight or flight. Amazing! This is very beneficial when there is a clear and present danger and this is a wonderful thing God provided for us to protect ourselves. Now remember, the memory is recording all of these things and in my little 6 year old brain that event was recorded accordingly-**Be afraid of all dogs!** And I was! As an adult I now know that dogs are wonderful creatures and very few are like the one I encountered. They bring such friendship and comfort to so many people including myself later in life. But it took rational thinking as an adult to 'rewrite' this opinion and create a new and rational memory. Sometimes our memory records things inaccurately which can be very dangerous. But in defense of our memory it is only recording what the brain is feeling and acting upon. That is why rational thinking is so crucial to learn in all circumstances so our memory can record accurate and reliable information to later rely on. I don't want to sound like I am oversimplifying things but truly, rational thinking is key to overcoming anxiety. I know this sounds very trite and you probably think you already possess this ability. I thought I did. Many of us have been anxious for a very long time and didn't even know it. Many of us have stored 'fake news' in our memory bank unknowingly while perhaps we were going through difficult times in our life. The great news is that all of this can be repaired through true self examination of our thoughts and memories. The 6 year old Gail put into her memory bank early on that all dogs were vicious and spent the better part of her adult life avoiding them completely. The adult Gail knows that this is not true and can remember the traumatic event but now can rationally come to a different conclusion. It takes practice, practice, practice. Whew!! I'm tired! But that's okay. Eventually this will be much easier to come by naturally and you can experience peace like you've never known before.

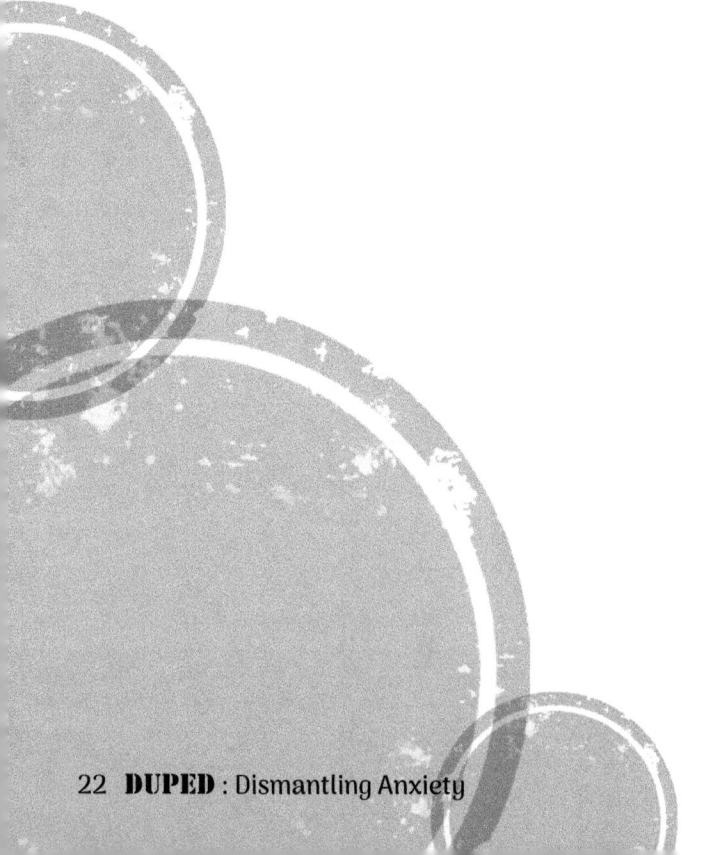

TRASH TALK #1

All or Nothing Thinking
Perfection or Failure

E ver try to fold a fitted bed sheet? **RIGHT**. It's fricking impossible!! For those three of you out there who somehow have avoided performing this maniacal task let me enlighten you. The fitted bed sheet, unlike the wonderfully smooth top sheet, has gathers at all four corners. Sometimes these gathers have elastic in them to make them even more laborious. Great when they're resting nice and snug on the bed. Nightmarish when coming out of the dryer and needing to be folded and put away in the linen closet. I have one friend who refuses to have more than one set of sheets so she doesn't ever have to fold it. She washes it and puts it right back on. These gathered corners make it literally impossible to fold without wrinkles. Maddening to all of us who fall in this category of thinking--perfectionism. All or nothing.

Remember Monica on the TV sitcom Friends? Everything had to be just right. Nothing out of place. Neat, orderly, organized. Perfect. Well, I am Monica. Yes, that would be me. And that's great, until it's not. Trying to be perfect often pushes you into anxiety or prevents you from ever starting anything for fear of failure.

We've all heard the phrase "Beauty is in the eye of the beholder". Well, so is perfection. Perfection is very fluid and fickle. Perfection doesn't recognize the color gray. It's all black or white. Perfect or Failure. In rational thinking, striving for perfection is very motivational and oftentimes produces revelations of improvement when perfection is not attained. But for those with anxiety, failure at perfection only produces more anxiety.

"Don't compare yourself to others. You will never end up on top." Another nugget from my friend, Jan. In my quest for perfection I always compared myself to others and guess where I **always** landed?!! On bottom! I have missed out on so many wonderful things in life simply because I was too afraid of failure. Too afraid of not being perfect. So sad.

Have you ever noticed that God always used imperfect people in the Bible to accomplish incredible things? His Will? People like Moses, who actually murdered a man who was beating another man. He lost his faith at times and was angered. Moses screwed up on a lot of things. Many scholars also believe that Moses had some sort of speech impediment. But God picked this man to carry out a monumental task. And you know why? Because God didn't make **PERFECT** people!!! Isn't that a relief? It should be! But it also shouldn't be used as an excuse to not try our best and be productive either. Striving for excellence to the best of our ability should be our goal.

Yes, my friend. I am a fitted sheet. And so are you. I am thrilled! Know what my new favorite color is? You guessed it!! **GRAY!!** Oh, I still love the **word**, Perfect. Use it all the time. I aspire to it but I don't let it control me or define me anymore. My definition of Perfect is no longer someone, something or someplace without any kind of blemish. I can't tell you how wonderful it is to be free of this anguish. **Perfect.**

TRASH TALK #2

Labeling

"Sticks and stones may break my bones but words will never hurt me". Remember that childhood chant? Don't you wish it were true? Words have pierced the souls of many, leaving an indelible scar. Changing the course of people's lives forever. Words can be weapons if not used responsibly and rationally. You cannot "unsay" something after it has been said. Only apologize. And sadly, for some, hurtful words will never be erased from their memory thereby forming a lasting, often damaging opinion of themselves.

It's funny how you can do something and never even realize it until someone else points it out to you, isn't it? It was probably on my second visit with Jan that she asked me this question, "Why are you so mean to yourself?" I've told you before I was brutally honest with Jan and spoke freely and frankly with her just as you do with yourself. According to **ME**, I was stupid, dumb, useless, lazy and a burden and embarrassment to my family. Whew!! Who needs enemies, huh?!!! This was one of the first things she pointed out to me and it was true. This was how I saw myself and labeled myself on a daily basis. In reality and retrospect I now know that I am **NONE** of those things. How did this happen? Anxiety. Wow.

Jan put a stop to all the negative name-calling immediately. I had no idea it had done so much damage to me. I had done it for so long and it came so effortlessly. Every time I had called myself a negative name it took away more and more of my already minuscule self-confidence. I really had to work hard on this. Watch what I was saying internally to myself. It took practice to not be mean to myself. Every once in a while, when I would slip up, Jan would look at me, grin, and say "I see mean girl is still alive and well!"

Today I do **not** call myself names or label myself. When I make a mistake, I acknowledge it, try to correct it and go on. I also try very hard to enact this attitude and assumption about other people as well. Very important! **YOU** are your best advocate.

I feel like I didn't dwell long enough on this subject because the gravity of it is so great. The advice sounds so simple but truly you will find it difficult to correct this negativity. It will not be easy. It will take time and lots of practice. Please do not dismiss this part of your recovery. As trivial as it may sound to you and give you thoughts of 'skipping over', I urge you not to do that. Please take this as seriously as everything else we've talked about, because it is. You **can** be self-disciplined, which is admirable and our goal, but kind to yourself at the same time. This builds self-confidence and self esteem.

"No one can make you feel inferior without your consent."

Eleanor Roosevelt

Exactly!!!

TRASH TALK #3

Jumping to Conclusions
Mind Reading/Fortune Telling

I don't mean to brag **but**, I am soooo good at these two things, mind reading and fortune telling, that I should probably charge a fee for my services! I can tell you just what you're thinking. Even when you're not. And who needs to consult a palm reader, crystal ball, Tarot cards or Astrology with this kind of talent? I can tell you anything you want to know. Just ask me. I should have my X-Ray vision any day now.

I'll bet right about now you're thinking, **"Really Gail?! Really?!! Hmm….I think not!"** And of course you would be right. Now who do you suppose gives me this kind of confidence that convinces me that I have these super powers? An anxious mind.

But isn't it amazing how many of us think we actually possess these super powers without even realizing it? How many times a day do we send a text message on our phone to someone and if we don't immediately get a return text we automatically think they are mad at us or are ignoring us. We have read their mind and made an absurd assumption. People are busy!! Some people lay their phone down and never pick it up until **they're** ready to use it! It simply is not the center of attention for everyone. I remember a while back a friend had sent me a text that I didn't know exactly how to answer back without fear of offending her so I procrastinated until I thought I could put together just the "right" words. In the meantime, I ran into her unexpectedly and apologized profusely for not returning her message and you know what her answer was? She said, "Oh, did I send you a text?" She truly had forgotten and couldn't even remember what it was about! All the while I had been sweating bullets and creating this scenario in my mind over what I thought she thought!! Thinking we can read other people's minds can be very dangerous and almost always inaccurate. My husband, Jack, is one of the most rational guys I have ever met. Proof positive that opposites attract, huh? But seriously, I can't tell you how many times he has said to me, "Gail, I can't read their mind" in answer to a question I **know** he couldn't know for absolute because indeed **he** is not a mind reader either. What we're really talking about is assumption or opinion, not fact and we should all extend this grace to everyone.

Fortune telling with an anxious mind is very dangerous because it will usually propel the person to fulfill their pessimistic prediction. You have predicted failure before the journey has even begun. And because of this negative prediction the journey, task, event or whatever is being scrutinized has little chance of success.

It is best to leave the Super Powers to the people at Marvel, DC Comics and Hollywood. Animation and fantasy, unlike real life, can be drawn, erased and redrawn, written and rewritten, without any repercussions. Unlike Life.

Remember when I told you that Memory was the smartest guy in the room? Well, Habit is definitely the **strongest!!** He is Popeye the Sailor Man on steroids. (Just revealed my age, huh?) He is the WWF Heavyweight Champion of the world. Winner of every Tough Man contest. He is King Kong. He is Spandex! (Gotta have a sense of humor in all this!) In short, Habit will kick your butt!!

Habit and Memory keep us alive. They are our automatic pilot. They work hand and hand **but** Habit cannot exist without Memory. Period. Just like fire can not sustain itself without oxygen. You have to have a memory before you can have a habit. Habit is wonderful. We use it a million times a day without ever realizing it. But Habit is also a double-edged sword. I would love to say that all of our habits are good but of course we all know they are not. And once a habit is developed, good or bad, it is **VERY** hard to break. Ask anyone who has ever tried to stop smoking. Anxiety leads us to a lot of bad habits. So does OCD, Obsessive Compulsive Behavior. And then there are ANTS and NATS, both annoying as hell and almost as dangerous! (Steady Batman. Last acronyms, I promise!) ANTS are Automatic Negative Thoughts and NATS are Negative Automatic Thoughts. Same things. Anxiety wears us down and we become complacent and allow this dangerous talk to become our Self Talk. We start to see everything in a negative way because remember, anxiety is FEAR. After a while, negative thoughts become Habit and we don't even realize they are negative because Habit feels normal, doesn't it?

Negative thoughts are not rational thoughts. Negative talk is Trash Talk. Anxiety taught us this discourse.

Who doesn't love the Property Brothers on HGTV? Or Chip and Joanna Gaines on Fixer Upper? They take broken down, outdated homes and make them absolutely beautiful! Before you think I've wandered out into left field here, please stay with me. I'm going to give you a visualization technique. On both of these television shows they take a property that at one time was a new build but over time has become in disrepair, usually through neglect or lack of maintenance. Your brain is your house. God deeded your brain to you when you were born. Over time things happened. Life happened. Some things maybe not so good. Instead of contacting the Property Brothers or Chip and Joanna Gaines to help renovate your house you mistakenly hired a guy with no scruples, Anxiety. The first thing he did was give a guy named Amygdala the run of the house. Remember this guy? We've talked about him before. Hair on fire, screaming misfortune at every turn? Yeah, that guy. Seriously, this guy has a very important job but his room in your house should be about the size of a small broom closet. He needs to stay on the thin side. He does not need to overeat. He thrives on fear. He devours rational fear **and** *imagined* fear. He cannot tell the difference. It **all** tastes like chocolate to him! So, as your anxiety grows so does your amygdala. He no longer can fit in the broom closet where he was designed to fit. So you start tearing down walls to make more room for him. He gets bigger and bigger with more and more control. You are at his beck and call. Pretty soon he **owns** you. The negative thinking has become Habit and fed the amygdala. But remember, **you** own the deed to your house. It will take work, time, self discipline, faith and practice but YOU can starve the amygdala and put him back in the broom closet where he belongs. **Still** a much needed item in your house but at the right proportion. Rational thinking creates good habits. Pray for it.

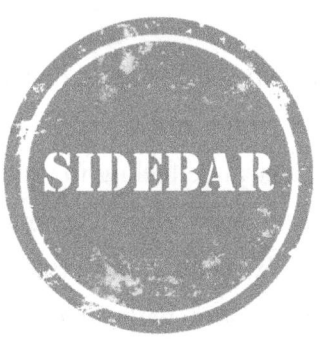

Okay boys and girls, go put your barnyard boots on. Today we're going to walk in some **deep** doo-doo and I don't want you to ruin your good shoes. Wow. This is going to be very difficult for me to talk about with you. Not because I am ashamed of what I'm going to tell you but when I reflect back on this time it absolutely terrifies me. **But**, it also qualifies me to have our next conversation because I have personal knowledge of it. I've been there. It is not going to be hearsay. This is my experience. I absolutely hate it when people give you advice that they have zero personal experience with. Talk to me when you have walked in my shoes. I am very cognizant of this and try very hard to be sensitive to a subject that I have no personal knowledge of. I can't tell you how badly it hurts to have a parent tell you "they know just how you feel" when you have lost your child and their child is standing right in front of you. Back off.

When I first sat down to have this conversation I didn't think I would venture into this, but it is a very integral part of my story, so here goes.

On November 4, 2016 I took a flu shot for the very first time in my life. I was 62 years old. God had always blessed me with good health, other than genetic high cholesterol, which medication and exercise took reasonably good care of. Never had I entertained the idea of taking a flu shot. I had recently seen a commercial on TV about how important it was for senior adults to get the flu shot and

I really liked and trusted the celebrity that was doing the advertisement so I did it. Amazing how easily we can be influenced, isn't it? 13 days later I noticed a strange feeling in the balls of my feet that stayed with me constantly. A few days later my ankles felt like they would not hold me up. My balance was getting wacky. On Thanksgiving night I was trying to shop with my daughter-in-law and I had to lean on the shopping cart to make it. I went to my doctor, who I love and trust, and he did every blood test imaginable. My autoimmune test came back with very high numbers but couldn't pinpoint the culprit. I continued to get weaker and weaker and started losing weight. I went to many specialists and Guillain-Barre syndrome was suspected but was never confirmed. This syndrome damages the nerve cells, usually starting in the feet or legs and travels up. This syndrome has been associated with the flu shot vaccine. Now, I want to stop right here and say something very important. I am **not** against vaccines. They are hugely important in saving lives but like any medication there are risks involved. Every person has a unique metabolic system and for the majority of people vaccines are very safe and effective. Unfortunately, I believe I was not in the majority. Clearly, vaccines prove more of a risk than a benefit for me. At this point in time we are nearing (I pray) the end of the Covid 19 pandemic. Vaccines have been very controversial and political. It is very sad. Okay, enough about vaccines. I just wanted you to know what my experience was that led me to the medicine cabinet that I alluded to when we first started talking. Remember me telling you about the rabbit hole I fell in that was so deep that even Bugs Bunny himself would be racing for the medicine cabinet? Well, this is the experience that got me there and held me captive for a very long time. On a trip to the emergency room, soon after my initial symptoms began, I unfortunately had a doctor who prescribed me Xanax. I am sure this doctor did not mean to harm me in any way. I am a grown adult and take full responsibility for my own actions. I had **never** taken an anti-anxiety drug in my life. I didn't have it filled immediately but a week or so later when my health continued to spiral downward with no answers I went to the pharmacy and had it filled. Worst decision of my life. Poor Bugs. He didn't know what hit him. For the next year and a half I bounced off and on, more on than off, Xanax and Klonopin with a short stint of an antidepressant and sleep medication to boot. The Xanax and Klonopin made me a zombie. And a mean one. My anxiety went to the moon! I couldn't take it PRN, meaning 'as needed' because I needed it all the time! I took it every 4 to 6 hours and the dosage kept getting higher and higher. When I tried to get off of it the withdrawal symptoms were so unbearable I would go back on the drug. I was addicted. The hole I had dug for myself was so deep I could feel the flames of hell licking at my feet. My legs were getting better, thanks to a wonderful physical therapist, but now I had lost control of my mind. Now let me stop right here and say this. I am **not** against anti-anxiety drugs. They have helped countless numbers of people. I was just not one of them. When I finally went to a psychiatrist to try and get well she insisted that part of her treatment plan was to see a therapist. I had no choice, so I did. Best decision of my life. A good therapist can help you with the underlying issues that cause your anxiety without the side effects of a drug. That's a **HUGE** plus and certainly worth the effort!! Praise be unto God, my wonderful family and friends, I have been drug free for five years. I will never forget how happy I was when I could finally cry and feel love and emotion again! Now I want to reiterate again, I am not against anti-anxiety drugs but without exploring the reasons as to why your chronic anxiety exists you will never be well. Anti-anxiety drugs have absolutely no medicinal value whatsoever. Zero. None. They are a sedative and nothing more. I wanted them to take all of my problems away but sadly they only created bigger ones. Finding

Jan changed my life. She told me on the very first visit that she hoped we would be a "good fit" but only time would tell. I was very blessed to get a wonderful, patient, compassionate, Christian therapist right off. I wanted to be well so badly I did everything she asked of me and most of the time didn't feel like it. (Remember, I'm a rule follower) I was brutally honest with her and confided information to her that I have never told anyone else. I trusted her implicitly. She never lied to me. She slowly brought me out of the rabbit hole and put my feet on solid ground. She gave me self confidence which I never had before. She taught me how to love myself **and** forgive myself. She gave me tools to think rationally which is always a deterrent to Anxiety. Turns out I have been anxious all of my life. I really knew that but never wanted to admit it. I had always been a perfectionist with OCD, a people pleaser. Then I suddenly lost my teenage daughter in a car accident and when my health was on the line it was just too much. I broke. Into a million pieces. Then the anti-anxiety drugs took me to a depth of low that I didn't even know could exist. Life happened to me just like it does to everybody else. I don't think **anyone** puts Anxiety on their "Bucket List" of things to do before they die. It is what it is **but** you **can** change it. That beautiful, powerful piece of property that God deeded to you at birth gives you the power to change it.

You want to know what absolutely blows me away?!! The fact that even today in the 21st Century most people are **still** more socially accepted taking medication for anxiety than those seeking counsel/therapy. We claim to be such a sophisticated, forward thinking world but still are so antiquated when it comes to mental health. Therapy or counseling seems to be far more accepted when it's a celebrity or sports icon. Many athletes seek what we call 'sports psychologists' and benefit greatly from it. These athletes know that all the athleticism and talent in the world can only take them so far without good mental health. I cannot take credit for this next sentence but it is so true. "The most common way people give up their power is by thinking they don't have any." Seeking help for anxiety and cognitive distortions is still greatly stigmatized and keeps people from living their best life to its potential. So sad.

Anxiety is fear. What are you afraid of? Getting better? Dig deep. Confront your demons. Cultivate rational thinking which grows self confidence and independence. Remember the last scene in the movie The Wizard of Oz? The Good Witch tells Dorothy that she has had the power to get herself back to Kansas the entire time of her long, arduous journey. The red ruby slippers she was wearing the whole time held the power to get her back home. It's time to take off your barnyard boots and put your ruby slippers on. The truth will set you free.

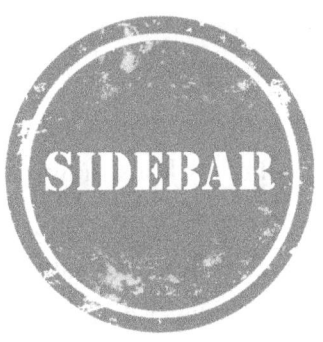

"**P**ray for rational thinking". Jan repeated those instructions over and over to me, week after week, month after month. **"What in the world is she talking about?!!"** I would say to myself. I **do** think rationally!! All I heard was blah, blah, blah…. Whatever!! Then one day the thought occurred to me, "If you're so rational Gail, why are you rotting away in this rabbit hole?" I had no idea that the rational thinking I was praying for was such a valuable gift and so elusive. I was so far removed from it, I couldn't even recognize that I didn't possess it. Ok, stay with me on this. Remember Spock from the television series Star Trek? Spock was half-human and half-Vulcan, remember? Spock was **THE** most rational thinking guy EVER!! You know why? He didn't possess any **EMOTION**. All of his actions and behavior was ruled by logic. Poor guy. He may have always made rational and logical decisions but I would hate to live without emotion!! Emotion is a wonderful God given gift that helps shape our personalities. Emotion gives us the ability to feel love, joy, fear, anger. It gives us energy and can rob us of it as well. Emotion can be tender and volatile. Quite the oxymoron, huh?! The Bible gives us many examples of Jesus's emotions. John 11:35 says "Jesus wept". In this scripture Jesus shows the love He had for his friend, Lazarus, and the grief at hearing the news of his death. In John 4:1-42 is the story of the encounter of the Woman at the Well. Jesus shows compassion in a great way to a woman who was looked down upon in society. Jesus shows anger in Matthew 21:12-13 as he overturns the tables of the moneychangers set up in the temple. And for absolutely **all** of us Jesus shows us forgiveness in Luke 23:39-43 which is the conversation between Jesus and the thief on the Cross hanging beside him. Even in agonizing pain Jesus showed forgiveness. Emotion is a big player in our thinking and because we are human we unfortunately sometimes let our emotions act on our behalf first and rationale second. But, I want to add something here. Just because we think and act rationally doesn't mean we're not ever going to make mistakes. We definitely are going to make mistakes!! But rational thinking helps us not to repeat them. We can enjoy the beautiful gift of emotion but we must employ rational thinking with it. When we don't, there can be consequences that can last a lifetime not only to ourselves but often to innocent people. Luke 12:48 tells us "To whom much is given, much is expected." Emotion acts quickly and comes with responsibility and self-discipline. It's bred by spontaneity which is what makes it so wonderful! We don't want to be like Mr. Spock or a zombie but we can't let emotion alone make our decisions. This leads us to Trash Talk #4.

TRASH TALK #4

Emotional Reasoning

Ever hear of spatial disorientation? Me either. According to the National Transportation Safety Board this is what the late John F. Kennedy, Jr. was experiencing while he was piloting his small but very powerful aircraft that dove head first into the Atlantic Ocean on July 16, 1999. It claimed the lives of all on board, Kenndy, his wife and sister-in-law. Very sad. There were a lot of factors contributing to the crash such as darkness and haze. It is reported that in situations like this, pilots **MUST** rely on their instruments because they can have **illusions** that make them unable to accurately determine how the aircraft is moving. Again, it is **imperative** they rely on their instrument panel for correct and accurate data to keep the aircraft flying safely. By all indications it appears that Mr. Kennedy did not use or trust his instruments to right the plane, so in his mind, he felt like he was taking the plane in an upward ascent. He was not. Instead, the plane was actually making a downward descent with great speed plunging into the ocean. Spatial disorientation.

Anorexia Nervosa. I had never, ever heard this term until Karen Carpenter, famous singer/songwriter of the 1970's died on February 4, 1983 from a heart attack resulting from many years of suffering from this disease. She was only 32 years old. So sad. When she looked at herself, her illusion was one of an overweight person, not the frail, skeletal woman she actually was in reality. She felt fat and acted upon it, denying herself of food and nourishment needed to sustain her life. After many years of this abuse her wounded body could no longer comply.

The key component in both of these sad stories is the word **FELT.** One acted upon a feeling that tragically took his life and two others in a matter of minutes and another acted on a feeling that took years to rob her of her life. Both acted on how they *felt.* Their perception. Sadly, both of these tragedies could have been avoided. These were highly intelligent, successful people. They did **not** have a death wish. They had everything to live for.

Turns out our feelings aren't always accurate. They can betray us, confuse us. WHO KNEW?!! Anxiety does and this is part of his deceptive arsenal. This kind of Trash Talk is called Emotional Reasoning. How many times have we heard and maybe even made the statement "I went with my gut feeling" or "I can feel it in my gut". Those kinds of feelings that prompt us into taking a course of action without rational thought behind it are very dangerous. Feelings are fueled by emotion. I know they feel so very, very right, so obviously they **have** to be true. Right? Wrong!! And the longer we allow inaccurate feelings to go unchallenged the stronger they become.

Anxiety is a bitch. It robs us of our self-confidence and self-worth forcing us to rely on emotional reasoning instead of rational thought. Anxiety's job is to thwart rational thought. I think of the small, crying child clinging so tightly to the abusive parent, so afraid to let go because it's all the child knows. So sad. But we are not children anymore. You have a choice. Use it.

TRASH TALK #5

Overgeneralizing

Seeing a single negative event as an endless pattern of defeat

Who doesn't love WD-40? Introduced in 1953, it claims to be in 4 out of 5 households and has literally thousands of different household uses for this product. It acts as a lubricant, rust preventative, penetrant and moisture displacer. The name of this product is an abbreviated form of "Water Displacement, 40th formula. Notice something very interesting? The 40th formula means it was the 40th **attempt!!!** It took the inventor 40 tries before his now very successful product made it into your garage! Just think if he would have given up after 10, 20, 30, 35, 39 tries? He never gave up on himself or his product even after defeat.

How many times do we put the handcuffs on ourselves after we experience even **one** defeat, much less 39?! Anxiety loves a loser. It will give you every excuse to quit. It will console you with the words, "Well, at least you tried". It will lull you into passivity and render you into hopelessness for any future endeavors.

Life is all about Research and Development, my friend. We are all equipped with talents and gifts. Problem is, we just don't always know what they are. That's what Research and Development is all about. Anxiety tells you to be afraid to invest in research of any kind for fear of failure, ridicule and disappointment. What Anxiety is really afraid of, is you finding confidence in yourself and casting it aside.

I once expressed a fear of developing a hereditary condition that one of my parents was suffering from with the doctor that was treating them. I told him in dismay that I had a 50 percent chance of developing it. And he quickly came back and said, "Gail, you also have a 50 percent chance of **not** developing it." All of a sudden the playing field had been leveled for me with his words. I could now see the glass was half **full** instead of half empty. You know what his words did for me? They changed my **PERSPECTIVE.** Very important word in your quest for freedom from anxiety. Have you ever tried on a pair of prescription glasses that were not your prescription? So blurry you couldn't see anything clearly? That's exactly what anxiety does to you! It changes your perspective to a negative prescription and alters reality which thwarts confidence, optimism and productivity.

Research and Development can open up many doors that you were too timid to even try. Buy stock in yourself and invest boldly.

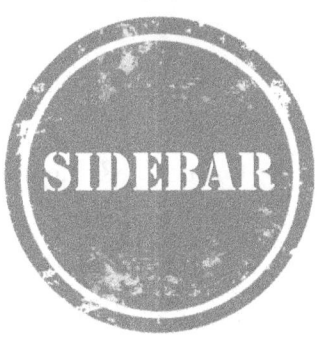

There's a new word, or term, floating around called "Influencers". This term is typically thought of as only being characterized to celebrities, athletes, politicians, social media voices, bloggers, etc. These are people that can "influence" how another person thinks or feels by their words or actions. Remember when I told you earlier that I took a flu shot for the first time in my 62 years of life simply because I saw a celebrity on TV promoting the flu shot for older individuals? I did exactly what she advised simply because I trusted her and her advice. And this is a person that I have never even met nor know ANYTHING about other than I thought she was a good actress and she was about my age. See how easy a person can be influenced?!! Happens all the time. But I have a News Flash for you. **We are all influencers!!** If you are living and breathing on this planet you are an influencer. Let me tell you this little story and you'll see what I'm talking about.

I am a very social person. Even with anxiety. I love people and love being out and about among people every day of my life.

One day, a while back, I was feeling particularly happy and light-hearted when I woke up. You know how some days are just better than others. Anyway, I had a spring in my step, a smile on my face and a song in my heart. I wanted to share my joy of life with everyone that day. Got out of bed, got myself ready and went to breakfast. Felt like a rainbow was following me. Glorious. **Then it happened.**

I ran into Oscar. Now, in full disclosure, Oscar is not this person's real name. The reason I call this person Oscar, is because this person reminds me of "Oscar the Grouch". Remember the furry little green muppet on Sesame Street? Lives in a trash can? **Not** a happy camper. Always sees the negative. Hence the name, Oscar, the **grouch**. Well, this person is Oscar in human form and was in particularly rare form that day. By the time we parted company I could barely put one foot in front of the other. All of my beautiful energy, joy and enthusiasm for life had been drained from me. I was no longer skipping and singing in my psyche. I was drooping and bent over. And then it hit me….Oscar had just sprayed me with RoundUp. For those of you who are not familiar with gardening, let me tell you what this is. RoundUp is a pesticide that is used to kill out weeds and grass. It is very powerful and effective. After being applied, whatever has been sprayed typically begins to droop and then die. Just like me. Oscar's negative words had penetrated and begun its mission. To destroy and kill. Mission accomplished.

I told you that story to enlighten you about how easily we can influence people. But there is also a bright side to this story. Ever hear of Miracle Gro? It too is used in the garden. It is a wonderful fertilizer, filled with nutrients that enrich flowers and vegetables that make them prosper and grow to their most desirable potential. Sprayed with this wonderful, life giving ingredient, they will stretch tall to reach the sun. Love it!!

We are **ALL** armed with RoundUp and Miracle Gro at our disposal. Every time we encounter another human being, whether it is in person, email, social media, telephone, letter, whatever form it is, we are going to spray one of these two powerful entities onto and into the individual you are in contact with.

So, my friend, how will you use your influence today? On others **AND** on yourself? You have two choices, RoundUp or Miracle Gro.

Think about it. It's so easy to become like Oscar. I know I am guilty of it myself many times, regretfully. But we **CAN** do better now that we are aware. Let's use Miracle Gro every chance we get and keep Oscar in his trash can with the lid **CLOSED!!!**

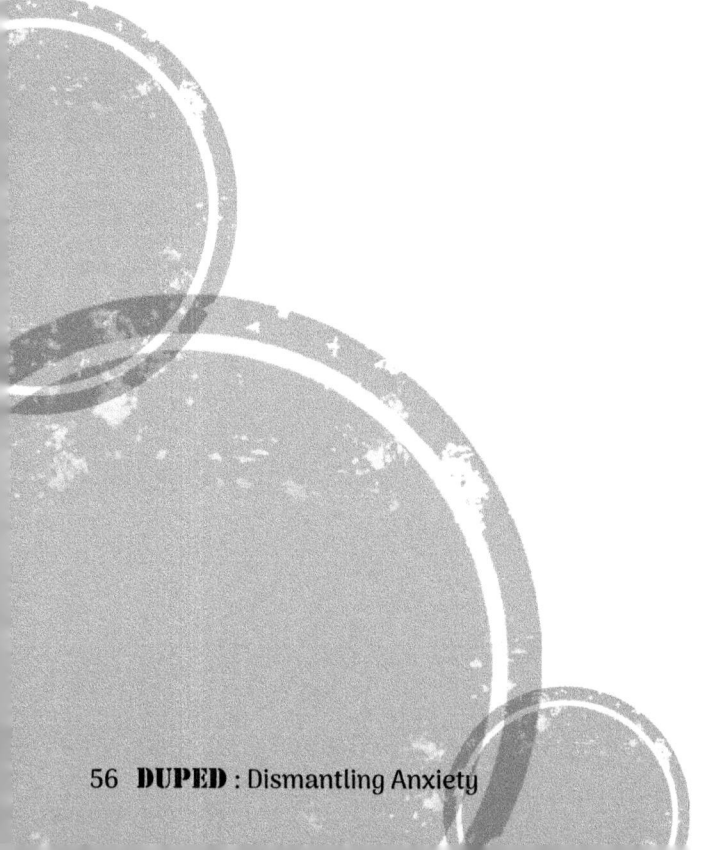

TRASH TALK #6

Personalization

"This is my fault".

G uilt is a very heavy load to carry and unfortunately, irrational guilt weighs just as much as the real thing. The mind uses the same bathroom scale to weigh them both.

For as long as I can remember, even as a young child, I always felt responsible for **everything**, even when it was totally out of my control or responsibility. I have no answers as to why this is, I just know that's how I always felt. Growing up I was never given undue responsibility and always felt safe and loved. But in my mind I always wanted people to be happy and safe and somehow or another I felt like I had to make sure that happened. That it was my responsibility. And when it didn't, I blamed myself. That is a heavy load to carry, my friend.

I want to introduce you to my daughter-in-law, Brittney. Now stay with me. I promise I'm not changing the subject. Brittney is the mother of three of my four wonderful grandchildren. She has a masters degree in physical therapy and is a very busy gal. She desperately longed for children and it took a while for her to conceive but when she did, **LOOK OUT!!** She had our first grandson in 2008 and in 2009 delivered a set of twins!! So she had 3 babies in diapers at the same time. Can you imagine?! This girl had to prioritize her time, schedule and responsibilities with surgical precision. Her plate was BEYOND full!! I was in amazement at how quickly this girl could go to the bathroom! Rival any guy! She did everything at warp speed to take care of her precious babies and did it wonderfully.

One day we were talking about something that I thought she would show great concern for, all the while knowing it was not her responsibility, and her reply were three words that I had never in my entire life strung together in a sentence in my head before, much less uttered out loud. They were: **Not my problem**. What did she say?! Could this be true? Could she possibly be right? Could the happiness and safety of the Universe not be my problem? Has my brain been misinformed all this time? **Whoa.**

Now I want you to know Brittney is kind, loving and very compassionate. I love and respect her greatly. She would do anything to help anybody but she is very rational and that has worked to my advantage! Her saying those three little words resonated with me significantly and shifted my way of thinking into a rational realm that has relieved me of much anxiety. Over the years I have watched her guide and instruct her children to be thoughtful, strong, caring, independent, rational thinking human beings. She has given them such an advantage in life with these invaluable tools.

Facing failure is difficult enough to bear when it is genuine. **Don't** let a misguided sense of responsibility rob you of your peace and lead you down a road without any "off ramps". Think it through. Remember, anxiety couldn't care less about the truth. It detests it.

Now there is also a flip side to this coin. Don't blame others for **your** mistakes. Sounds simple enough, doesn't it? The ADULT thing to do. **But**, anxiety loves scapegoats and will provide one for you every time. Free of charge, or so it would appear. We all make mistakes and rational thinking gives you the confidence to understand this, improve from it and offer forgiveness to yourself and others. The blame game can cripple you. Anxiety perpetuates it. Reprogram your thinking and moving forward will be your great reward.

TRASH TALK #7

Mental Filter

Never seeing our successes, only our failures

I love movies. I especially love the whole "movie theater" experience. The HUGE screen, the darkness, loud surround sound that you can actually feel and of course, the popcorn. Gotta have the popcorn! It's truly one of the only places I can actually lose myself and focus on what is before me. In 1990 one of my favorite pictures of all time came out. Partly because it was so good and partly because my then 14 year old daughter, Jamie, and I went and saw it together probably no less than 4 times. I so loved spending time with her. It was a great movie starring Julia Roberts as a beautiful prostitute named Vivian and Richard Gere as a very wealthy, smart, successful, handsome business man named Edward. In the movie, Edward meets Vivian on the street and takes her back to his hotel room. VERY fancy hotel room. Instead of it being what we call a "one night stand", they actually fall in love during the course of the movie.

It's funny how you can hear or see something that resonates with you immediately and stays in your memory for the rest of your life. It's THAT impactful to you. It has been 32 years since I first saw the movie and the dialogue I am about to show you I can still repeat to you verbatim. Vivian's words could have been my words at any point in my life. I still have to stave them off. Listen…

Vivian: *People put you down enough, you start to believe it.*

Edward: *I think you are a very bright, very special woman.*

Vivian: *The bad stuff is easier to believe. You ever notice that?*

How sad. Edward, of course, would never notice that because he would never have felt that way. He is a confident man. Comfortable in his own skin. He recognizes his failures but uses the knowledge gained from them to propel his successes.

I have spent most of my life being the one putting myself down, not other people. I needed no enemies. I only saw my failures and lamented them so grossly there was never room for successes in my mind. The bad stuff was ALWAYS easier to believe whether it was true or not. This was part of the reason at 62 years old I broke into a million pieces. I can't and won't live like that any longer.

I love the statement, "Most people are running from something that isn't even chasing them". That's what Anxiety does to you. It steals your self confidence and will not allow you to see any of your successes. Believe me, my friend, you HAVE successes. Take bold inventory and you will see them, just as others do. Learn from your failures to make greater successes. I recently heard the statement, "It's only a mistake if you don't learn from it". Valuable advice. Self confidence breeds success. Put it into practice.

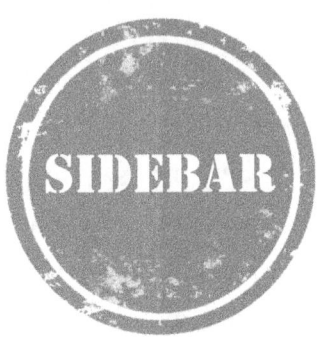

You want to hear something that would be very funny if it weren't so sad? Up until 5 years ago I truly believed that I was the only person that had bad thoughts. True story. Not making this up. I was so ashamed I, of course, never talked to anybody about it, thinking I was the only one. That kind of thinking stole 62 years of my life. So sad. This is where I would put an emoji with the little face filled with tears streaming out of both eyes.

I will never forget when I read these next words in a piece of literature about anxiety and OCD for the first time.

Everyone has unwanted or unpleasant thoughts sometimes; it's normal.

Just thinking about something won't make it happen. For example, if you think about winning a multi-million dollar lottery, it doesn't mean it will really happen.

Thinking a bad thought does not mean you are a bad person. It also does not mean that you want to do anything bad.

Oh My Gosh!!!! Is this really true?!! Could this somehow be a misprint?! I could not wait until I could talk to Jan to verify it's validity. **Hallelujah!!!** It was true!! I felt as if God himself had opened up the cell door of the prison I had locked myself into many years earlier. Thank you Jesus.

Incarceration for so many years had made me very weak. My mental muscle had not been exercised for so long it had begun to atrophy. And of course anxiety shows up for work early everyday and goes home late. Now the real work was about to begin.

Anxiety wants you to believe that you have no control over your thoughts or how you can react to them. He uses Habit to convince you of this. Anxiety is the one that tells you that every thought that falls into your head is by your own cognition and deserves deep examination, especially the disturbing ones. Those are the ones he wants to convince your brain are worth focusing on instead of taking them to the trash bin where they belong. **This** is why practicing rational thinking is so important.

I love analogies, parables and visualizations. They help me tremendously in retaining information. I have recently created one in my mind that has helped me alot with the "taming" of unwanted thoughts. I've named it "Unbridled Thoughts". Here it is. I hope it will help you as it has for me.

I love horses. I think they are the most beautiful animal God created. I love to hear their hooves pounding the ground when they are running and make that unmistakable sound that is in all the Western movies. Okay, as much as I love the horse I also recognize that man governs the horse. I "visualize" myself on top of the horse with the reins of the bridle in my hand. In my visualization the horse is my "thoughts", good and bad, right and wrong and my brain is the rider on top of the horse. When a bad or incorrect thought occurs and the horse starts bolting forward and wants to break into a full out run at top speed hitting every branch in our path, I pull back on the reins as hard as I can for as long as needed to make it come to a stop. The horse (thought) doesn't like it. He doesn't want to stop but I am the master and it is up to me to stop it by pulling hard on the reins causing the bit in the horse's mouth to halt him. The horse (thought)

can be unruly and stomp his hooves and in some cases be so out of control will rear up on his hind legs and try and buck the rider off. The rider (brain) has to be very firm with the horse (thought) and not let the horse take control. After a period of time and repeated pulls on the rein, the horse will realize who has control and give up it's antics. The horse succumbs to the realization that the rider is the master and he is governed by such. After that they get along beautifully because the horse and the rider know their positions. I love it when I can visualize
the rider letting the horse run at full speed, making that beautiful sound with their hooves because then I know a beautiful, creative, productive, memorable thought is in progress. Rational thinking is the best food you can feed your horse. Happy Trails!!!

I sincerely hope I didn't lose you in this. Visualization is not for everyone but it helps me alot. My whole point in telling you all of this is that **you** are the one who gets to decide what thoughts you keep and what goes in the trash bin, no matter how relentless they seem to be. Anxiety will tell you you're not strong enough. That is a total **LIE**. It takes patience, forgiveness, hard work and perseverance but wouldn't it be so great to be able to govern your thoughts? **YOU** make the decisions and not anxiety?

I want to leave you with a quote that I love from Martin Luther. I hope it will give you food for thought and put a smile on your face as well.

"I cannot keep the birds from flying over my head but I CAN keep them from building a nest in my hair!!"

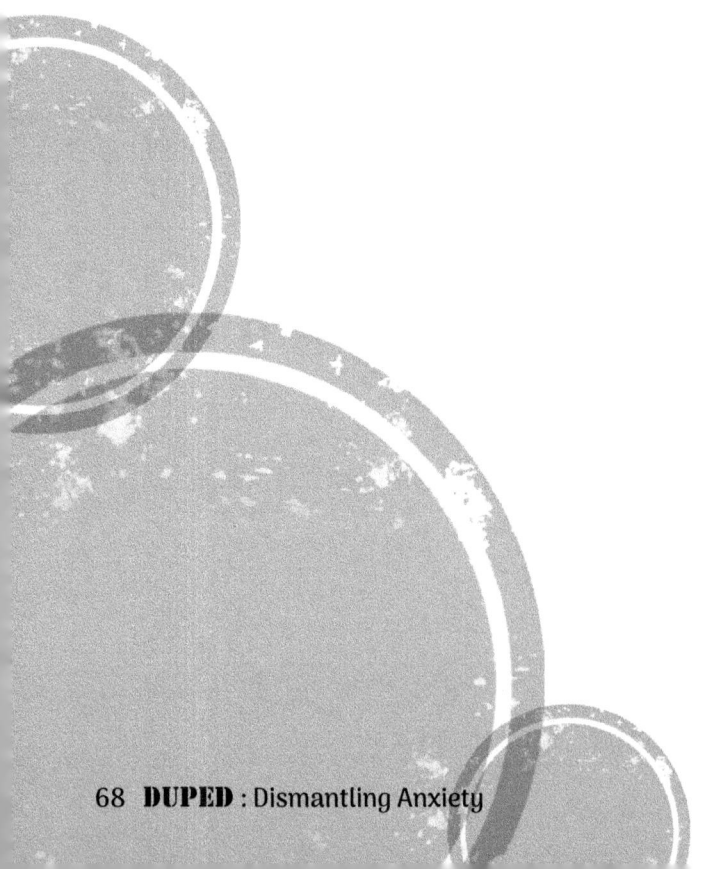

TRASH TALK #8

Disqualifying the Positive

D o you remember the day that you put on that zebra shirt, aka referee shirt, and started calling all the plays in your life as penalties? Out of bounds, holding, roughing the kicker, off sides, pass interference, targeting, DQ? **You** became the referee that everyone hates!! The one that called the legal touchdown back and took the points off the scoreboard without even looking at the playback! Please forgive me for all the football metaphors but it's almost Super Bowl Sunday!! Poor timing for this conversation for all of you non football enthusiasts. Please forgive me but hopefully you get my meaning.

Somewhere along the way we started only recognizing all the negative things we've done and totally ignored any of the positives. When we lose our self-confidence and self-esteem all we can see is the negative.

I had done this **BIG TIME!** I couldn't even gracefully or graciously accept a compliment from others. It was as if I had to talk them out of it. That whatever form of adulation extended to me was totally incorrect. Remember the notebook Jan had me bring to our sessions? She addressed this kind of Trash Talk right at the start. For two weeks she had me write down everything I did from the moment I woke up until I laid my head on the pillow at night. EVERYTHING had to be written down from showering, putting my makeup on, fixing my hair, getting dressed, going to breakfast, shopping for groceries, paying bills, doing laundry, exercising, preparing dinner, cleaning the kitchen. Everything counted.

Turns out getting dressed is a pretty big deal after all! Who knew?! I didn't. Maybe you didn't either. Anxiety loves to trivialize anything you do that is meaningful as menial and mundane. Its job is to devalue our self-worth. I have seen this happen to many people who are transitioning from one Season of Life to another.

I have recently observed this happen to a wonderful guy. He is transitioning from public life to retirement. Before retirement he was **THE** guy whenever he walked into a room. Everyone wanted to be close to him and have his ear. He had a title in front of his name. Now I cannot even begin to imagine how difficult it must be to go from being the center of attention in a room to being asked if your name is on the guest list. It was as if all of his former accomplishments in life were the only thing of value and anything beyond or after that was of little or no relevance. But you know what? It took a little while for him to adapt to his new life but he now realizes he is still **THE** guy to the most important people in his life--his family. His new accomplishments after public life may not be in the news media anymore but he realizes they are just as valuable.

The truth be told, we are all in an "identity crisis" from the moment we are born, simply by transitioning from one Season of Life to another without ever even realizing it. And all of these Seasons come with their losses but also with their gains, if we will only accept them graciously. But the bottom line is, we all want to remain and **feel** relevant. And that, my friend, is not a bad thing.

Learn to accept a compliment graciously, my friend. Learn to **give** yourself compliments when you deserve them. This builds confidence and perpetuates rational thinking. You can only be as successful as you allow yourself to be.

TRASH TALK #9

Should Statements

Using the words 'should', 'must', 'ought' to make you feel Guilty

Remember good 'ol Stretch Armstrong? He is a large gel-filled, toy action figure made of latex rubber. He was shaped as a short, stocky, muscular man with blond hair and wore black wrestling trunks. He could be stretched by his four limbs from his original size of about 15 inches to 4 and sometimes even 5 feet! He could hold this enormous stretch for a short period of time before shrinking back to his original shape. He was introduced to the world in 1976 by the Kenner Toy Company.

Well, in 1976, my son Shane, was five years old and of course Stretch had to come live at our house. Oh, he loved pulling Stretch to his full capacity! Over and over and over, which was great, until one day Stretch could take no more and red gel started to ooze out of him. Stretch had met his Kryptonite at the hands of an adorable five year old little boy!! Poor Stretch. Lost all his Super Power!

How many times a day do you do this to yourself? And for how many years? You viciously berate yourself with verbal abusive language like "I **should** or **must**", usually said in an effort to keep pace with someone else. We compare ourselves to what we see on the outside of an individual and what we don't realize is they are letting you see only what they **want** you to see. This is called "window dressing". You cannot see the interior of the heart or the home. NO ONE can do it all. SOMETHING or SOMEONE suffers. Just like Stretch with his gel oozing out of his body, you too will 'bleed out' if you constantly compare yourself and stretch yourself to be something that truly doesn't even exist--Perfection, or more accurately, our perception of it. We wag our finger at ourselves with accusatory statements that are unrealistic and unattainable.

Please don't misunderstand what I'm saying here. I am a HUGE proponent of hard work, grit and perseverance. These are the very attributes that give us progress in every field of life. I pray that these would be considered descriptive words of myself. I admire and applaud all of these characteristics. I think competition is great. It helps us reach our potential. But somewhere along the way we have begun to reach for the World's opinion of what is admirable rather than being true to ourselves. We chase after images that have been "airbrushed" by the artist's hand to appear flawless. We look at lives that have been "photoshopped" and try to conform to it. All this does is produce more anxiety. So sad. I recently watched an old Western movie the other day on TV and there was this farmer who was perfectly happy in his life doing the same thing every day, taking care of his crops and livestock. He was totally satisfied, content and happy. Another man came along and convinced him that his life on the farm was very mundane and boring and he should go into town and experience something new. Reluctantly, the farmer went with him into town and long story short, the farmer got shot and killed. Now the moral of this story is NOT to persuade you or scare you into avoiding new adventures but rather what struck me was this farmer's total contentment and satisfaction with his life right where he was. He felt happy and fulfilled. Contentment, Satisfaction….Don't ever let anyone rob you of this very rare and very valuable gift. Treasure it.

Please, do not conform to the "ever changing" world and its ideas of perfection. Stretch to be the best YOU. Be true and kind to yourself and repetition of these will develop confidence which is toxic to anxiety.

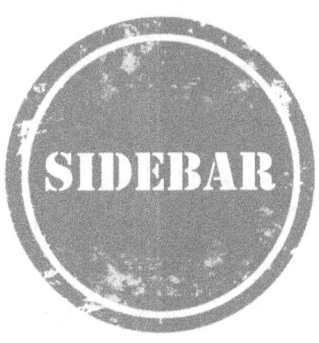

I didn't want to talk about this, but I know I have to. Obsessive Compulsive Disorder (OCD), the purest form of Anxiety. I want to make something very clear. Just because a person has Anxiety **does not** mean they have OCD but every person who has OCD **has** Anxiety.

I am very thankful that our society has become more enlightened and accepting of this vicious disorder. But maybe it's become a little less enlightened and a little too accepting. So much so that it's almost fashionable to say that you have OCD when in fact you truly don't. People have come to associate OCD with perfectionism only. So who doesn't want to be considered perfect? It's true that perfectionism is one of the **many** characteristics of the disorder but certainly not the defining characteristic.

Let's dissect these words and see if you still consider yourself to be OCD. Okay? Obsessive means excessive, often to an **unreasonable** degree. Compulsive is used to describe people or their behavior when they cannot stop doing something wrong, harmful or **unnecessary.** They are compelled to complete some sort of ritual to cleanse the thought process. Disorder is self explanatory. Still want to be fashionable? Didn't think so. I will never forget a conversation I had with a friend one day who was convinced that she had OCD so naturally I took her at her word and believed her. We began to talk and as I related to her the seriousness of my compulsions I could see this "deer in the headlights" look overtake her face. I knew I was in trouble. She was absolutely shocked at hearing my struggles with this demon, OCD. I was embarrassed and felt betrayed. Yes, she was a neat freak, a perfectionist and germ conscious, but she quickly realized she did NOT have OCD.

OCD is a very seriously haunting disorder that disrupts and ruins lives. It sucks. People who truly have OCD do **not** want it nor did they do anything to acquire it. It is still a mystery to everyone. People who do not have this disorder may say, "I just don't understand it!" Well guess what? We don't understand it either. So how about a little grace? For those of you very fortunate ones who have now been diagnosed with negativity of this disorder, go grab a Snickers candy bar and take a break. You can skip over this part of our conversation. Come back in a few minutes. See you in five…

Okay, now we can talk. If you are like me you have probably tried to hide your OCD behavior for as long as you can remember. It really is a good thing that people are letting their guard down, especially famous people that others admire, and admitting their vulnerability to this disorder. No, we are not crazy or dangerous. For a very long time I accepted my fate and tried to work around it. But no more. I am now armed with information that changes the playing field. OCD gives you a suspicious mind which in turn gives you the "What if?" Syndrome….**assuring** you that trouble, turmoil and strife are lurking around every corner. You know the drill. Anxiety **LOVES** people with OCD. We're his favorite appetizer. He chews us up and spits us out depositing us into the Land of Dread. But you don't have to take up citizenship there. You **can** escape this captivity with the power, **practice** and discipline of rational thought. OCD is irrational thought mixed in with a healthy dose of **FEAR**. I am learning to manually OVERRIDE these irrational thoughts and stifle the compulsive behavior associated with them. I'm not going to lie to you. It's hard work and it takes time. It's not a quick, easy fix. But the more times you override these thoughts and compulsions you create a new memory of living without them. Then what happens? Remember? You have created a new Habit. A new habit without OCD being involved!

I know OCD has you fearful that if you don't complete these compulsive rituals that something bad will happen. Believe me, I know the incredibly powerful hold this feeling can have on you. It translates into your whole body and you just finally give in to the rituals because it's easier to, than to withstand the fear mounting in you if you don't. Well, I'm here to tell you I haven't exploded yet and I'm working on this every single day with great success. When I fall down, and I do, I don't let it negate all the progress I have made.

I care deeply for you, my friend. I want you to know that you **can** get better. Life is harder for you and me because of OCD but we are armed with life saving information now that we can implement into our lives and way of thinking. Don't give up. I'm not.

Okay guys, we're through now. You can come back in. Hope you enjoyed your candy bar.

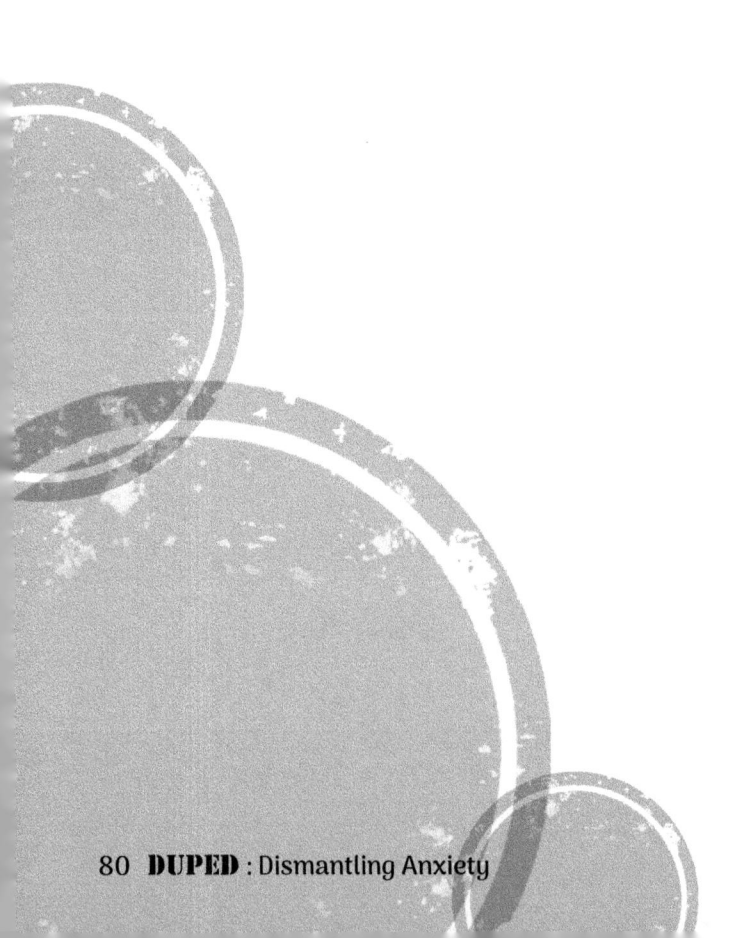

TRASH TALK #10

Magnification and Minimization

Catastrophizing and the binocular trick

Ever look at your face close up in a magnifying mirror? It can be your best friend or your worst nightmare!! I have one of these little beauties mounted right on my bathroom wall next to my sink. Use it absolutely every day to put my makeup on and for several "teeth checks" during the day. Up until very recently we had gotten along pretty well. One morning I was putting on my makeup as usual and happened to take a long, hard look at my nose for some unknown reason. "Hmmm……Looks a little bit different this morning" I say to myself. "Maybe bigger? Is that it?" SO, the more I looked, the bigger my nose got! "Oh my gosh!! My nose has grown overnight!! What has happened to me?!! I'm hideous!! I can't ever leave the house again!!" True story! I kid you not. I had worked myself up into such a frenzy I became paralyzed with fear. That's what Anxiety does to you. **Totally** irrational thought. **Of course** my nose had not grown overnight. BUT my little daughter-in-law recently told me that as we age our noses and ears get longer! Yikes!! Gravity is great until it's not, huh? And, by the way, I now think they should put Warning Labels on magnifying mirrors saying that they "may cause anxiety!!" Right?!

Seriously, it is so easy to blow things out of proportion and behave inappropriately, regretfully so. Chronic anxiety keeps us on edge and brings out the Amygdala in our brain (Remember the little guy we talked about earlier? Hair on fire, screaming the sky is falling?) to make us leap into irrational thinking. Suddenly we are viewing everything through the magnifying glass making situations or mistakes appear larger, worse, dangerous or more significant than they really are. And then what do we do? We act upon this **mis**information.

Anxiety can lead us down the opposite spectrum of this as well. We tend to minimize our good qualities or accomplishments rather than building upon them. If we can teach ourselves to recognize our accomplishments that will build our self confidence to beget even more. I know this one is a lot harder to do for most of us because self confidence can be in very short supply when you have anxiety. One step at a time, one building block at a time. Put the binoculars down, my friend. Practice rational thinking and you can view your life with fresh eyes.

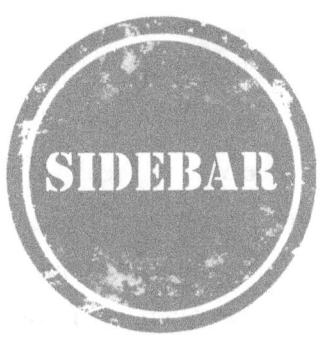

Do you know how many times the words, or some form of it, "Do not be afraid" is written in the Bible? 365 times. I don't believe this is a coincidence. I believe God knew we would need to be reminded of this every single day of our lives.

Fear is much like a weed. It pops up out of nowhere, grows quickly and spreads in every direction devouring everything good in its path. Constant, chronic fear will eventually turn into Anxiety. It's a done deal.

We're nearing the end of our conversation and I find myself grappling for words to bring this next subject up. Weird, huh? Maybe because it's so important. So, here we go.

You're going to need some help with this. Fighting fear and anxiety. More than I or anyone or anything on this earth can give you alone. I don't care how high your IQ is, how much money you have, how strong you are or what position of influence you have attained in this world. This, my friend, is above your pay grade.

I'm not going to preach to you. That is not my job or the reason for our conversation. Perhaps you already know Jesus Christ as your Savior but for those who don't, this is a big deal. He wants to help you. He loves you. He wants you better.

Now for those of you who are looking for a Genie who will grant your every wish or some sort of Biblical Santa Claus, He's not your guy. The two greatest gifts God gave us are (1) Salvation through

Jesus Christ and (2) Free Will. I find it pretty amazing that someone would give their only Son to die in agony on a cross for our sins and then give **us** Free Will. Free Will is a really **BIG** deal. Never take it for granted. Free Will gives us choices. You can choose to accept the wondrous gift of Salvation or you can choose to reject it. The choice is totally yours as are the consequences of your choice.

Okay. I feel better now. I, personally, cannot imagine my life without the hope, comfort, love and dependability of God. He is my Fortress. Enough said.

John 3:16 "For God so loved the world that He gave His only begotten Son, that whoever believes in Him should not perish but have everlasting life."

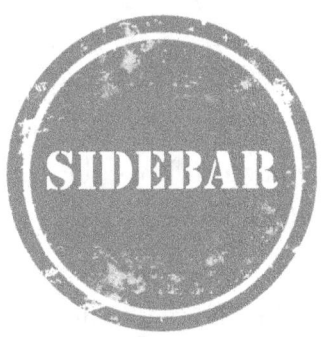

ENCOURAGEMENT. Okay, stop right there! I see your hand, poised, ready to turn the page. You have this subject covered, right? No need to stop here and dwell on something you already know, right? I know this from experience, remember? Now, please, put your hand down, lean in close and listen to me very carefully… **You're going to need this skill.** I promise, it is invaluable to your recovery. Sadly, but realistically, Anxiety has removed or erased any trace of this skill when it attacked you. You will literally have to **retrain** your brain to get this skill back online. I'm talking about learning to encourage **yourself** without the assistance of another human being. Recovery **cannot be maintained without this skill**. It is imperative that you learn how to be your own personal cheerleader, **especially** when the stadium is void of any fans and you are totally alone.

Now any counselor/therapist worth his or her salt will tell you that the entire goal of counseling is to get you to a point of living on your own without their help. To arm you with tools and skills to combat the psychological damage that Anxiety has done to you. The goal of any type of counseling is to one day be independent and no longer need their services. I remember the last day of my counseling sessions with Jan, and I didn't even know it at the time. It had been almost a year since I had visited with her because of Covid. I was so excited to see her and talk with her. We had a great reunion. At the end of our time together I made an appointment in a month to see her again. On my drive home, (I live quite a distance from her office) I realized I hadn't asked her any questions. I had taken my notebook (remember what a good student I am!!) but had not written anything down. By the time I reached home I realized I had and could continue to live on my own. Jan had instilled in me a self confidence that I truly had never known before in my life. She had given me tools and skills that had gone untapped and for the first time in my life I felt like a strong, independent adult with reasoning power. **WHOA!!!** I thought about this revelation for another day or two and then texted Jan and canceled my next appointment. She was elated also! Her student had graduated!!

One of the most important tools in encouraging yourself is the act and art of forgiveness to **yourself!** You're going to screw up and make mistakes in life. We all do. The rational thing to do is to forgive yourself, make a mental note not to repeat the mistake, make amends if need be to the injured party and MOVE ON. It's that forgiveness and MOVE ON part that is difficult for us. Anxiety takes the event and plays it continuously on a revolving loop in our brains draining us of time and energy. A few days ago this very thing happened to me. It robbed me of almost 24 hours of the beautiful gift of Life! I am sorry to say it took me that long to shake it off and resume rational thought, forgiveness to myself and self encouragement. It takes **practice, practice, practice.**

Encouragement is such a badly needed nutrient in ALL of our lives. We need to be able to encourage ourselves and others as well. I want to tell you a little story real quick about two frogs. One of the frogs was totally deaf. They were walking together one day when they fell into a deep, deep hole. Of course they immediately started trying to jump their way out by using their powerful legs. When word got out about the misfortunate mishap of the two frogs the entire Frog community immediately responded by encircling the hole and peering down at them. They watched as the two frogs tried tirelessly with all of their strength to jump out of the hole to no avail. After a while the other frogs above the hole watching started to throw their hands and arms up, waving and yelling down to the frogs saying, "Give Up!! You'll never get out of that hole!" After seeing and hearing this for a while the frog that was not deaf gave up trying and laid down and died. The other frog, the deaf one, just kept jumping and jumping and finally reached the top and was out of the hole! When he was safe, the other frogs asked him why he kept on trying when his circumstances looked so bleak. He replied that it was all of the encouragement that his fellow Frog community had given him! The frog could not hear what they were saying but believed in his heart and mind they were encouraging him to not give up by waving their arms and yelling! Perception wins every time.

The moral of this story is obviously to "never give up". But you will need **fuel** to accomplish this and it comes in the form of **encouragement.** Always have it at your disposal, for yourself and for others.

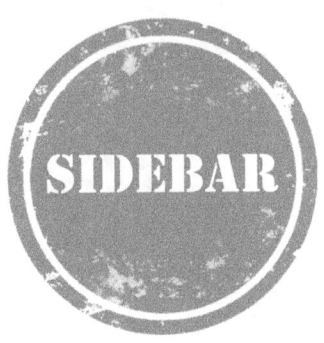

Overthinking. Doesn't sound dangerous, does it? It's just being cautious, right? Or is it? Is it caution? Or is it **fear?** The most harmful element of Overthinking is the very silent, very methodical erosion of one of your most valuable assets that God blessed us with, Automatic Pilot. There is a distinct difference between being thorough and overthinking. Being thorough comes to a conclusion. Overthinking does not. If left unnoticed and unchecked it can lead to something more debilitating such as OCD. Automatic Pilot enables us to accomplish everyday tasks without thinking or relearning them. Breathing, swallowing, blinking….all on Automatic Pilot. Works pretty good, doesn't it? Overthinking fills you with doubt, hesitancy and robs you of your self confidence. Overthinking is anxiety in action and becomes habitual. It can be corrected as can any bad habit. It will take time, focus and perseverance to overcome but well worth the effort. When conquered, your Automatic Pilot will re-engage as well as your self confidence which is the hallmark of a calm mind. Think about it. But not for very long.

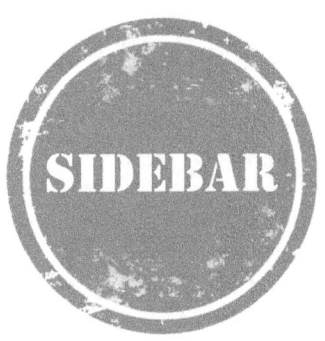

Okay. There is one final thought I want us to talk about before we say good-bye. It affects absolutely everyone on the planet, anxiety ridden or not. Hard to talk about, but absolutely necessary. So here goes.

The truth be told, we **all** have an "appointment" with death from the moment we are born. As we age, become ill or allow fear to become the controlling factor of our mind, we naturally think about death more frequently. **PLEASE**, don't get caught in Death's Waiting Room leisurely flipping through the pages of a magazine **waiting** for your name to be called. Make death **find** you!! Let him find you at the ballpark or the theater or dining with friends or shopping or at work or enjoying your favorite hobby or dancing or singing or helping someone in need. The list is endless and it's called Living Life to the Fullest!! It's time to turn off the fear faucet, my friend. Employ Carpe diem into your life…Seize the day! Let go of the words, "If only"…and look at the beautiful gift of life with grateful eyes. I don't care how old you are, your current situation or the medical diagnosis you have received. The Bible teaches us that no one knows the "appointed" time of our death, with the exception of God, and I'm pretty sure none of us fall into that category.

Life is full of "adjustments" and "alterations". **Don't let anxiety be your tailor.**

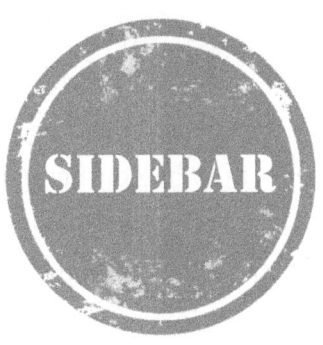

M an!! Just when I thought we were going to wrap this up, another thought pops into my head! I know some of you are avid, voracious readers and the amount of context here will probably not completely satisfy your thirst, perhaps leaving you longing for more. I'm sure many of you would describe the perfect day as having the time to curl up with a good book and read all day long. As for me, that scenario would be about as appealing as spending the day at an acupuncture clinic!! I'm a magazine girl. Meaning that however much context can be presented between the pages of a monthly subscription magazine is plenty for me! Isn't that funny?!! This may be all I have to give you for now but I promise we will keep in touch.

Okay. here goes. Don't you just hate it when someone tells you that your relationship with them is going to be on a "need to know" basis?! I **do!!!** Drives me absolutely CRAZY!! **And** being the sitting President of the "Control Freaks Anonymous" Club, I know this for sure! It blows!!

But here's the deal…Our relationship with God has **got** to be on a "need to know" basis. And you know what? It's for our own good. I'm sure your brain is telling you right now just how absurd and unfair that statement is. Been there, thought that. But let me tell you a true and very personal story.

I have two beautiful, wonderful children. A handsome, grown, adult son, Shane, and a beautiful teenage daughter, Jamie. I tried to

DUPED : Dismantling Anxiety

be the best parent I could be, like all parents do. So much so, that I was what they call in today's terms a "helicopter" parent. Meaning that they hover over their children, constantly trying to protect them and keep them out of harm's way. Okay, I can live with that.

On Tuesday, August 27, 1991, at about 12:30 p.m. I had a knock at my door. I was home on my lunch hour from my job. It was our local Fire Chief. He delivered to me every parent's worst nightmare. My 15 year old daughter, Jamie, had left the High School campus in a car for lunch with five of her favorite friends. They were involved in an auto accident on their return to school. My Jamie did not survive. I cannot begin to tell you how badly this hurts to this day. But that is not the point of my story. I told you all of that, to tell you this. I have had 32 years to think about this and I am convinced that had God given me a glimpse of what was about to befall my beautiful daughter, I would have totally screwed up the wonderful relationship Jamie and I had together.

Jamie was smart, fun, fearless, loving, kind, energetic, optimistic and absolutely bursting with life. It was all I could do to keep up with her and because she loved me and she knew how much I loved her, she tolerated my helicopter parenting but didn't let it slow her down! I'm SO thankful for that. I know myself well enough to admit that had I "known" what the events of that day would bring, I would have become a **DRONE** parent, snuffing out all of the beautiful, spontaneous times of life. The last time I saw Jamie was the morning of that horrible day. I was leaving for work and she was in her bathroom, doing her hair. We were laughing and my last words to her were, "Be sure and call me when you get in from school". "I will!" she replied. I did not receive a phone call from Jamie that day or any day since.

There is a song by Garth Brooks called "The Dance". It was one of Jamie's favorite songs. She played it repeatedly. I would hear the music wafting from her room until I could repeat the words verbatim. For those of you not familiar with the song I want to read the chorus that is so meaningful to me. When you have time, listen to the entire song. It is painfully poignant. Here it is:

For a moment
All the world was right
But how could I have known That you'd ever say goodbye

And now I'm glad I didn't know
The way it all would end The way it all would go
Our lives are better left to chance I could have missed the pain
But I'd have had to miss the dance.

I am so thankful for God's infinite wisdom and putting me on a "need to know" basis. Because of this valuable relationship, I didn't miss "The Dance" with my beautiful Jamie. We live with the consequences of our actions. Certainly, we are living with the consequences of Adam and Eve thinking they "needed to know" and we all know how badly that turned out!! Cultivating trust and faith in God will quench the sometimes insatiable desire for "needing to know" more.

Okay, I know I just gave you some pretty heavy stuff to think about in this big, long letter I have written to you. Thanks for staying with me to the very end. I have poured out my life, heart and mind to you because I care for you and want to help you through this difficult journey you find yourself on. I have let you look at every square inch of me and that's pretty scary! You know that unwritten rule that you absolutely **NEVER** look inside a woman's purse? Under NO circumstances?! Well friend, I just opened up my purse, turned it upside down and dumped it right out onto the kitchen table for your examination!! I am now challenging you to be very brave and do the same thing. Unzip that backpack, purse, tote, pocket, suitcase or whatever bag of preference that you carry your valuables in, and dump it out onto the table. I think you will be very surprised at what you will find. Anxiety is very sly and cunning. I think you will be shocked to find all sorts of "trash" that slipped into your bag when your back was turned. Anxiety is also a very skilled pickpocket. I think you will find a lot of your valuables missing. Things like confidence and rational thinking. It's time to take inventory of what has been stolen and dispose of all the negative trash that has made your bag so heavy. You can do this. I know you can. You have now learned the skills that give you the ability to separate fact from fiction. **Implement them.**

Proverbs 3:5-6

"Trust in the Lord with all thine heart; and lean not unto thine own understanding. In all thy ways acknowledge him, and he shall direct thy paths."

PARTING THOUGHTS

Remember good old recess? Elementary school? It was usually right after lunch and you were free to run all over the school yard and talk out loud to anyone you pleased. Do whatever you want. Unsupervised. Love recess!! I always think of the dreams that I have when I am asleep as my mind being on "recess", unsupervised by my consciousness. Free to roam anywhere I want. I will wake up some mornings and think "Why in the world did I ever dream that?!! I have NO IDEA where that came from!!" So, while your mind is on recess your beautiful brain is doing housekeeping chores. Things like storing new information, processing things, trashing useless information to make more space for relevant information. VERY important stuff. That is why sleep is so very important to our health. Mental and physical. Remember, your brain is an organ. Your mind is not. So, here's the deal. Listen closely….

YOUR MIND RUNS THE SHOW. Yep. True fact. But… it gets all of its information from your brain, correct or incorrect. And here's the kicker. Because of this, the brain has an advantage over your mind and rational thinking. The brain can be very persuasive and the biggest advantage it has over you is it also has control over your body. Remember me telling you earlier about the trip I made to the emergency room thinking I was having a heart attack? Turned out to be anxiety? Remember? Your body reacts to fear in all kinds of different ways. Muscle aches and tightness, headaches, trembling, heart palpitations, sweating, dizziness. You name it and an anxiety threat can do ANYTHING to you!! THAT is why rational thinking is so important. You have to let your mind control the body. Do not let your body control the mind. Your mind is the bouncer at the door. It can look at the thought entering and decide whether to let it stay or kick it out. Your brain doesn't hate you, as I once thought, it is only reacting to the information it has been fed. Fear silently crept into your brain short circuiting all your wiring. But the BEST news ever, is that it can be repaired! YOU possess the tools to do this! Your mind can override any lie or irrationality that your brain may give you. You have to use your mind to summon courage and self discipline to discern truth from untruth. We have just talked about many of these untruths. Remember all the Trash Talk we discussed? For a while it may seem as if your mind is playing ping pong bouncing the truth from the long held lies in your brain. But every time you score a victory, be very proud of yourself because I KNOW how hard this is. The reality is, we will always have anxiety in our lives. That is simply the cost of living. BUT God wired us with protective devices (Remember the Amygdala?) to handle it. We don't have to live with chronic anxiety that disrupts and robs us from the beautiful gift and joy of Life. I am fighting for you. I am praying for you. Without God…..all I can do is wish you luck. With God….Welcome to the Future!

Last thing. You **have** to have a Fight Song!! Being a former cheerleader I know this to be true!! You know what mine is? It's 'I'm Still Standing' by Elton John. I love it!! Find the one that is right for you and make it your mantra. There is so much more I wanted to tell you. Perhaps next time. Until then, it has been an honor, my friend.

Always, Gail

E ver been duped? I have. **BIG TIME**. I believed the lies that Anxiety fed me for the better part of my adult life. I followed the fear. Obeyed the commands. Know what Anxiety really is? It's fear gone rogue. Am I speaking your language? Time to put Anxiety on a leash. **A short one.**

Now, in the last words of one of the most courageous men that ever lived, Todd Beamer, passenger on United Airlines Flight 93, Sept. 11, 2001, as he and other passengers thwarted the attempt of terrorist hijackers to fly the plane into the US Capitol...**Let's roll.**

Gail Bennett Fry resides in Midwest City, Oklahoma with her husband, Jack. She continues to write and does motivational speaking. Gail's unique and very personal style of writing exposes her own human frailty and vulnerability forged with perseverance to overcome. She invites and engages the reader in conversation with her open and frank dialogue. Gail is also the author of "My Journey to Jamie: Revisited".

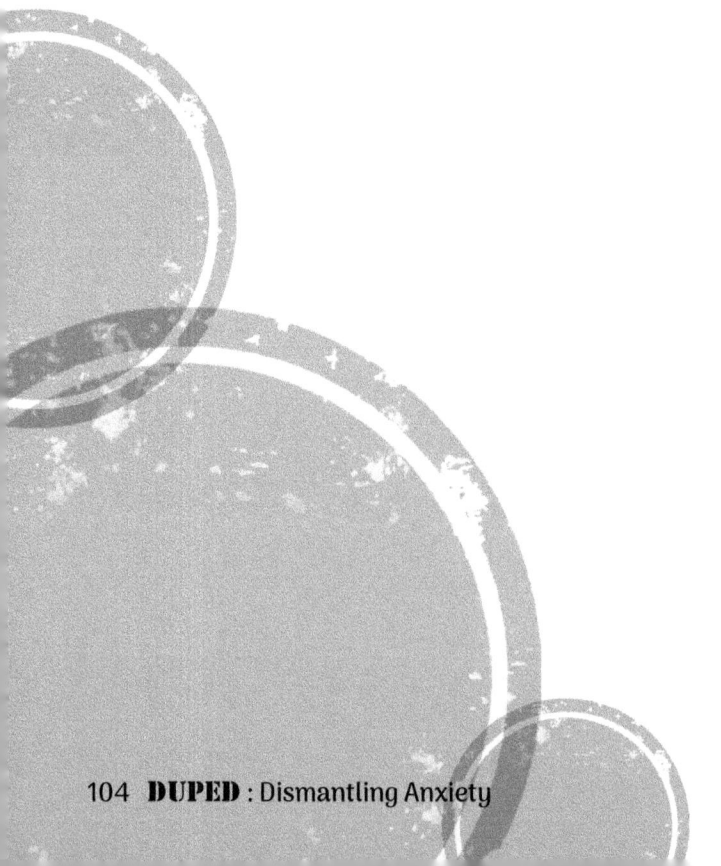

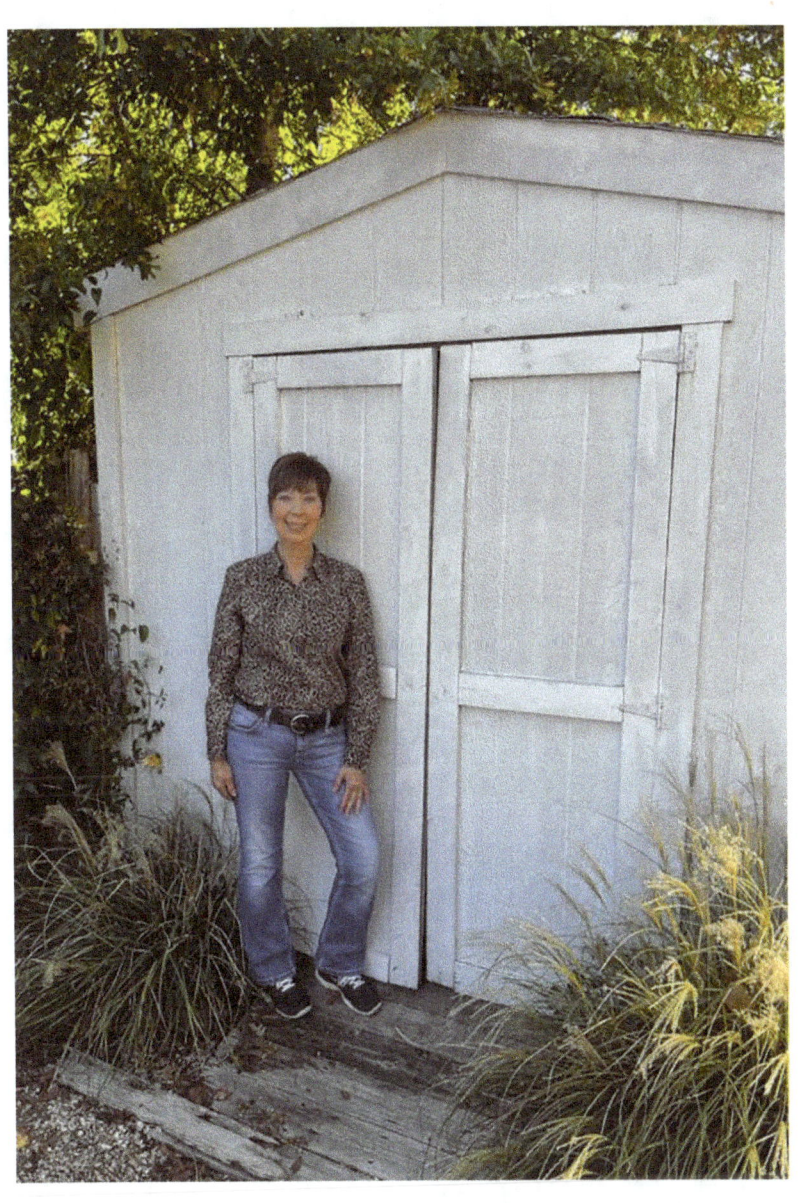

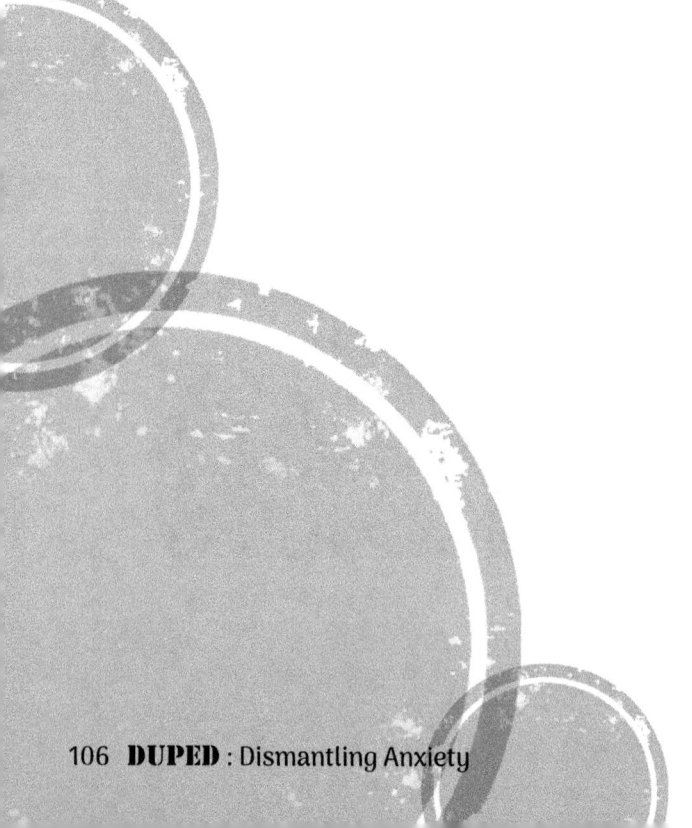

Reflections:

www.ingramcontent.com/pod-product-compliance
Lightning Source LLC
LaVergne TN
LVHW021120080426
835510LV00012B/1769